Paleo Diet
Good or Bad?
An Analysis of
Arguments and Counter-Arguments

By M. Usman

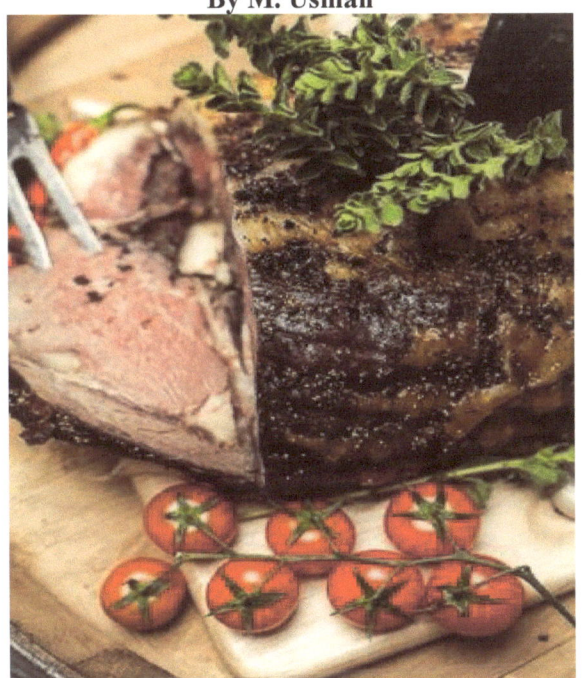

Health Learning Series

Mendon Cottage Books

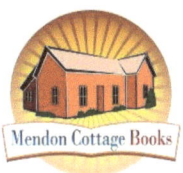

JD-Biz Publishing

Disclaimer

The information is this book is provided for informational purposes only. It is not intended to be used and medical advice or a substitute for proper medical treatment by a qualified health care provider. The information is believed to be accurate as presented based on research by the author.

The contents have not been evaluated by the U.S. Food and Drug Administration or any other Government or Health Organization and the contents in this book are not to be used to treat cure or prevent disease.

The author or publisher are not responsible for the use or safety of any diet, procedure or treatment mentioned in this book. The author or publisher is not responsible for errors or omissions that may exist.

Warning

The Book is for informational purposes only and before taking on any diet, treatment or medical procedure it is recommended to consult with your primary care provider.

Our books are available at

1. Amazon.com
2. Barnes and Noble
3. Itunes
4. Kobo
5. Smashwords
6. Google Play Books

Table of Contents

Introduction

Part I – A trip through time

Imagine yourself travelling back in time - far back. When you open your eyes, you are sitting on a small rock, about 10,000 years ago. The paleolithic era of history is almost at its end. Birds are flying around. There are trees and animals everywhere you look. The air is clean and so nice to breathe in. A cool wind is

blowing through your face. Suddenly you feel hungry and you know that it's time to eat. You call some of your fellow tribe members. Spears are brought out and after some chasing and running you all hunt down a bison. You take out meat from the bison's body and roast it on fire. Then someone brings in some natural herbs and berries from nearby and thus, a delicious well-balanced meal is served and everyone gets his share. Tired as everyone is after the hunt, everyone sits down to eat.

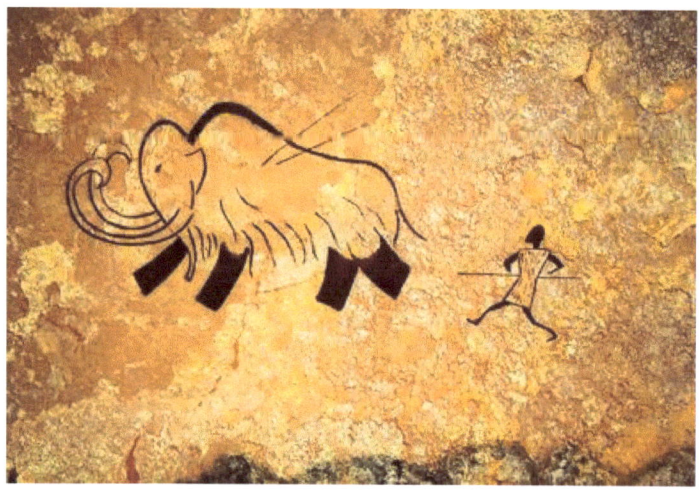

You look around. These fellows of yours have large muscular bodies. They are all tall and strong, with a large appetite. But what about you ? You aren't so bad off yourself. With huge muscles, you even surprise yourself with your strength. You never felt so fit and healthy in your modern time.

The old man continues : "They are a lazy people. They live only to eat and sleep."

Then the tribe leader calls out : "Men, listen ! Have you heard the stories?" Intrigued by his question, everyone else huddles around him. "No, we haven't. What are you talking about ?" one of them asks. "They say that there is a tribe in the north." he continues. "They use strange ways to get food. They bury small seeds in earth, then water them, and then after some months, from the place where they had sown the seed, food comes forth." Everyone is awed by this seemingly impossible thing. "What magic ! What magic !" cries one of the others. The tribe leader calls out "I wish that some of you go there and bring me that magic." But before he can say anything else, "No, you must not ! I have heard of them." an old voice comes from a corner. Looking around, you see an old man there, his face showing clear signs of age. The old man continues : "They are a lazy people. They live only to eat and sleep. But we! We run, fight and hunt, as our fathers did before us and their fathers before them. Our lives are tough but we are healthy, happy and content ; we are strong and proud. You must not indulge with them. You will soon see that this ease which these people have invented shall only bring suffering and death to us humans." Others don't listen to the old man. Soon, in order to learn this strange art, some of them go in search of the magic tribe that gets food from the earth. But somewhere in your heart you know that the old man is speaking the truth. However, before you can tell them anything, the scene fades away.

10,000 years later, you wake up in a bed wondering whether it was a dream or reality that you just experienced. You look out through the window. The atmosphere is so different from that paleolithic environment. Everywhere, there are tall buildings. The air is polluted. Food is abundant and delicious but doesn't satisfy the appetite. People of this age, are fat and weak. Hospitals are filled with sick people of all ages. This is our age : The era of modernity!

Can going back to the diet and practices of that ancient paleolithic era solve our problem. Was the old man really correct ? Is our new diet the culprit behind all the diseases that we suffer from ? Read this book to get the answers to all these questions.

"Today man is trembling on the brink of another dietary revolution which will return full circle to the place where he began." Voegtlin 1975

Part II : Paleo diet explained – Return of the caveman

Paleolithic era literally means "old stone age" (from paleo – old and lithic – stone). Paleolithic era extended from about 2 million years ago to 10,000 years ago. The diet of this age is called paleolithic diet or the stone age diet.

It was 1975, when a gastroenterologist Dr. Walter Voegtlin first proposed the concept that paleolithic or stone age diet is the best diet for human beings. In his book, **"The stone age diet",** he explained that humans have adapted for 99 % of
history, to the ancient diet of meat and wild plants. He considered agriculture to have developed relatively recently and that human beings aren't adequately adapted to foods produced by agriculture. He held this maladaptation to be the factor solely responsible for many diseases of modern age such as cancer, heart diseases and obesity. And so, he concluded that the best diet for modern humans is the ancient diet, high in proteins and low in carbohydrates, because human bodies are adapted to this ancient diet of the paleolithic era. He asked everyone to reject all forms of modern diet that do not conform to this criteria. In his own words:

"Today man is trembling on the brink of another dietary revolution which will return full circle to the place where he began – to his Stone Age diet of meat and fat." [1]

And in this way, the concept of paleo diet came into existence. Since then, several attempts have been made to exactly replicate the diet of ancient humans and to determine its efficacy. Many variants of this diet are now available. But all are based on the same purpose : "To find a diet that best suits the adaptations that humans have been undergoing throughout history." Thus, when the termed "paleo diet " is used now, it doesn't refer to the exact diet of human ancestors but to :

".... a modern dietary adaptation that attempts to mimic the diet of the paleolithic human." [2]

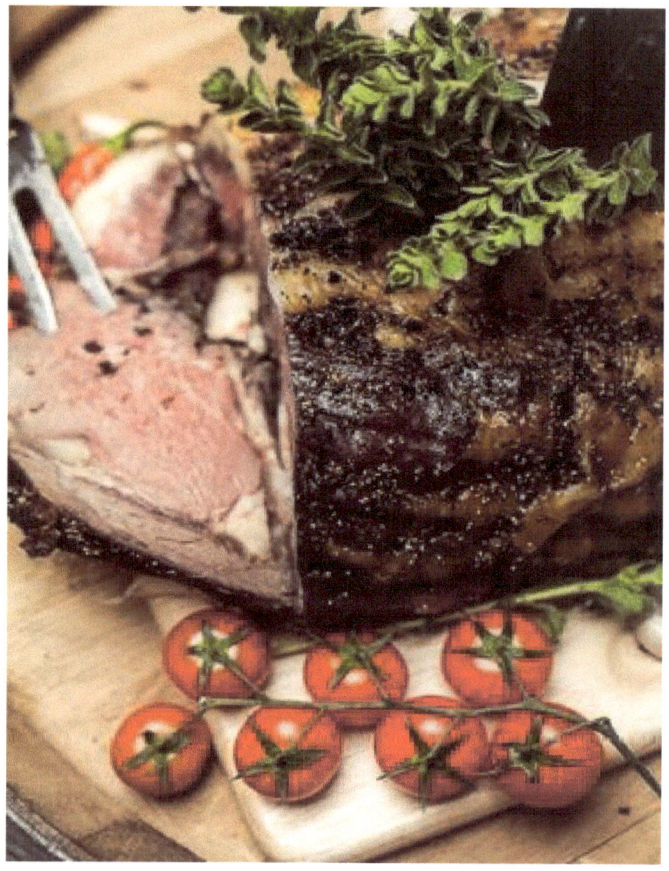

This modern adaptation or the paleo diet is marked by its high content of proteins and fat and low content of carbohydrates. Furthermore, several versions of paleo diet totally reject all foods that weren't available to the humans in that era including vitamins and dairy products. Despite many variations, paleo diets have several components in common. These are :

1. **Meat**: Meat is the basic component of almost all paleo diet programs. It is believed that human originally adapted for a carnivorous life style. And since his origins, he has been feeding on the meat of hunted animals.

   Furthermore, only meat of wild animals or grass-fed beef is allowed in paleo diet because grains and other foods, given to farm animals today, weren't available in the paleolithic era.

2. **Fish and other sea foods:** Fish and other sea foods are also a part of paleo diet. These are a rich source of proteins. As with the animals, wild fish is allowed in paleo diet. Farm fish is discouraged as it is fed on artificial foods.

3. **Eggs:** It is proposed that primitive humans also consumed eggs of different birds.

4. **Fruits and vegetables:** Wild fruits and vegetables are essential components of paleo diet. Paleolithic humans used to pick different fruits and vegetables from wild plants to supplement their diet.

5. **Exclusions from the diet:** All modern and processed foods are completely avoided in paleo diet plans. These include grains, legumes, salt, refined sugars, processed oils and dairy products.

So, a low carbohydrate content and a high protein content, in addition to avoiding modern processing and farming, characterize paleo diet. Some variations include intake of calcium, as calcium is deficient in most paleo diet plans. It should be noted here that the exact diet that paleolithic humans ate is unknown. The modern versions of the ancient diet are based on archeological evidence.

Since the popularization of concepts, numerous scientists have vehemently supported it while several others have gone against it. While some researches seem to support Voegtlin's theory, others have shown little or no benefit. Furthermore, certain logical questions have been raised regarding the validity of this diet. This book attempts to analyze all the arguments favoring and opposing the paleo diet, with an unbiased eye, in the light of modern research. References have been provided throughout the text. At the end, links to the pertaining research papers and books have been given so that interested readers can have access to further information. (see the References section at end)

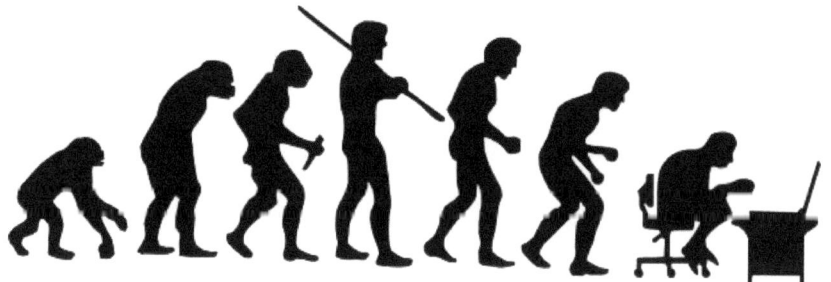

Section I : Arguments favoring paleo diet

Several scientists most notably Loren Cordain, Staffan Lindeberg and Boyd Eaton have researched and given much evidence in support of paleo diet. The basic argument favoring paleo diet is based on evolution: that humans have genomic adaptations for paleolithic diet and hence, a diet based on the stone age diet is best for humans today. Another point in favor of paleo diet is that humans, world-wide, are suffering from many diseases which seem to have dietary origins. These include, in particular, obesity and diabetes which are due to excess intake of carbohydrates. A return to the ancient diet of human beings, will not only eliminate all these diseases but also result in a healthier, stronger and fitter body. These arguments are explained, in detail, in this section.

Argument 1 : The genes of old

According to the theory of evolution, humans evolved from an ape-like creature called "Proconsul" about 2-3 million years ago. Humans developed an erect posture, an upper limb that could grasp and a higher intelligence. All these factors led to the superiority of humans over the other descendants of "proconsul" so that the other descendants became extinct. Humans thrived and built tools for themselves.

For around 2 million years, humans underwent continuous adaptations and evolutionary changes to support their paleolithic lifestyle.

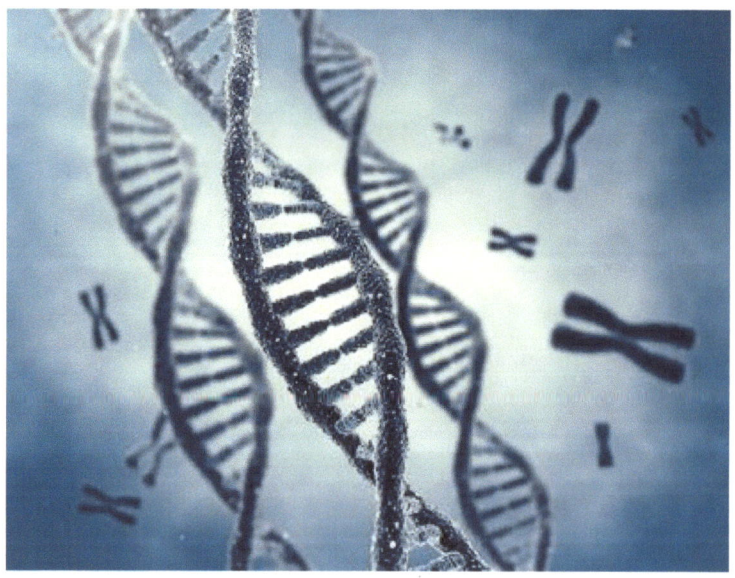

From 2 million years ago to 50,000 years ago, humans obtained food largely by hunting wild animals and eating their meat. Voegtlin considered these primitive humans to be purely carnivorous.[3] It was only about 50,000 years ago that they started to consume plants and vegetables. And it wasn't until 10,000 years ago, that agriculture became widespread and plants and grains became widely available, signaling the end of paleolithic era and ushering in the age of agriculture (the neolithic era).

During the long period from 2 million years ago to 10,000 years ago, humans underwent continuous adaptations and evolutionary changes to support their paleolithic lifestyle. However, since the advent of agriculture too little time has passed for humans to adapt to their new diet. So, the basic postulate behind evolutionary health promotion in general, and the paleo diet in particular is: The old genes of ancestors are still present in all humans and they are adapted to a largely carnivorous life-style. Boyd Eaton explains this point in the following words :

" ...particluarly since the Neolithic revolution of 10,000 years ago, cultural evolution has proceeded more rapidly than genetic evolution producing an even greater dissociation between the way we live and the way our genomes have been adapted to."
Boyd Eaton et al. [4]

The basic rationale for eating paleolithic diet is simply that it is better suited to   genetic makeup of human beings.

Argument 2 : Paying the price of modernity

The second argument supporting paleolithic diet follows from the first argument. The proponents of the paleo diet put the blame of modern diseases on diet. They state that human beings have not adapted to the diet they consume in the modern era. This lack of adaptation to the agricultural food that human beings suddenly started to eat about 10,000 years ago, is responsible for most of the chronic diseases that are present today. Going back to the way humans used to eat, is the only way to cure all the modern diseases. In the words of Boyd Eaton :

"This discordance fosters the chronic degenerative diseases that cause most morbidity and mortality in contemporary affluent nations."
Boyd Eaton et al. [4]

These diseases include the following :
1. **Cancer:** Cancer is one of the most common causes of death world-wide. It has been suggested that cancer is caused in part by modern diet. High carbohydrate index which is a characteristic of modern diet stimulates insulin, a growth promoter. Any cancerous growth is promoted by insulin. Furthermore, certain agricultural foods contain opiates, which interact with immune system and decrease resistance to cancer.

Going back to the way humans used to eat, is the only way to cure all the modern diseases.

Paleolithic diet, on the other hand, is richer in its antioxidant content than typical mediterranean diet. These are effective in reducing the chances of cancer.[5]

2. **Cardiovascular diseases:** Eating a diet rich in carbohydrates and saturated fat – a characteristic of modern diets - causes the blood cholesterol level to rise. This cholesterol deposits in the walls of small arteries and by decreasing the blood supply to the heart and brain can cause heart attack and stroke respectively. The paleo diet, in contrast, is low in carbohydrates and rich in proteins and unsaturated fat. It causes a decrease in the blood cholesterol level, preventing these cardiovascular accidents. This has been proven by a research by Gary Foster et al. who compared low carbohydrate and high carbohydrate diets in 63 obese individuals. They concluded that

"The low-carbohydrate diet was associated with a greater improvement in some risk factors for coronary heart disease." Gary Foster et al: A randomized trial of low-carbohydrate diet for obesity. [6]

3. **Diabetes:** Diabetes type II is a disease in which there is resistance to insulin, a substance responsible for lowering blood sugar. Diabetes is also related to diet. Consuming a high-carbohydrate diet can cause excess release of insulin from the human pancreas. This excess insulin, if present in the blood for a long time, results in development of resistance to its effects. This leads to diabetes. In contrast to modern diets, paleo diet is low in carbohydrates. This avoids the stimulation of insulin release and maintains the sensitivity of tissues to effects of insulin. All this prevents saves a person from diabetes.

4. **Auto-immune diseases:** Paleo diet has been shown to decrease the incidence of autoimmune diseases such as lupus erythmatosus and multiple sclerosis.

The assertion that paleo diet results in lower incidence of chronic diseases has been one of the main arguments in favor of paleo diet. Nowhere is it more apparent than in the Kitava research conducted by Staffan Lindeberg. In Kitava, Papua New Guinea, modernization has not occured. The resident people still obtain their food by hunting animals or picking wild plants. Staffan Lindeberg did several tests of the residents and concluded that even the older people of the island (age group 60-90) were free from chronic diseases such as stroke or heart attacks.[7]

Argument 3 : Fighting obesity - "They are a lazy people"

Obesity is one of the biggest curses of our time. More than 500 million adults worldwide are obese. Obesity is the major cause of cardiovascular problems in addition to several other health related risks. It is also largely dependent on diet. Following is given how the modern human lifestyle leads to obesity and how paleo diet can decrease it :

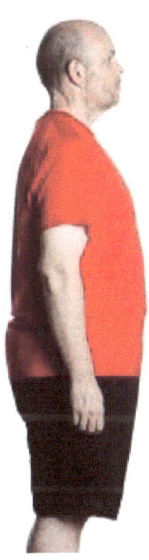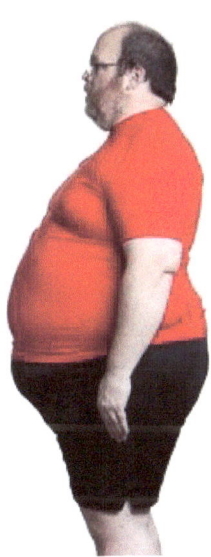

1. **Increased intake of fat:** Increased fat intake is related directly to obesity. The excess fat in a person's diet is stored in fat deposits beneath the skin, in the abdomen or around the kidneys. Especially dangerous in this regard is saturated fat. Although some components of paleo diet do include saturated fat, majority of paleo diet is free from saturated and rich in unsaturated fat.

2. **Increased carbohydrate intake:** Modern mediterranean diets and most other contemporary diets have abundant carbohydrates in them. People seem to believe that unless they eat plenty of carbohydrates, they will not feel satisfied. Excess carbohydrates, more than required by the body, are converted to fat and stored in a similar way as described for fats in the previous heading. All this leads to obesity. In contrast, low-carbohydrate paleo diet prevents excessive intake of carbohydrates and in this way, prevents obesity. Again, we refer to Gary et al who tested a low-carbohydrate diet in 63 obese people:

   "The low carbohydrate diet produced a greater weight loss (approximately 4%) than did the conventional diet for the first six months."

3. **Sedentary lifestyle:** The physical activity of modern humans is very restricted. So, when the old man in your imagination said : "They are a lazy people" he was quite right. Modern humans work, eat and sleep. Except athletes noone bothers to maintain even a moderate level of physical activity. This inevitably causes obesity because in such a case, even low intake of calories, exceeds the energy requirements and is stored as fat. Proponents of paleo diet, in addition to dietary changes, also recommend a high degree of physical activity to mimic the paleo lifestyle. This effectively prevents obesity.

4. **Satisfying appetite – Investing less, getting more:** It is a proven fact that paleo diet contains lower energy density as compared to modern human diet. For instance, a gram of Macdonald's sandwich contains approximately 2.4 calories per gram in contrast to 0.8 calories per gram contained in natural plants and berries, which are components of paleo diet. So, for the same amount of food and same amount of satisfaction, paleo diet offers less energy which decreases the chances of overeating and in this way decreases obesity.

Argument 4 : Healthier, stronger and fitter – The case of athletes

"What?" you may ask here, "I've been eating those delicious sandwiches and burgers ever since I remember. But, I'm still healthy. So this is all a hoax, right?" Unfortunately, however, while the modern diet may keep you going, it will never allow you to achieve maximum health that you can achieve. To achieve maximum health that you are capable of, you must take a diet that is most suited to your genetic makeup. In the words of Boyd Eaton :

"As a rule, biological organisms are healthiest when their life circumstances most closely approximate the conditions for which their genes were selected."

Boyd Eaton et al. [4]

"What?" you may ask. "But, I'm still healthy. So, this is all a hoax right?"

Furthermore, paleo diet is perfect for athletes who want to achieve maximum fitness. Athletes, due to their high level of physical activity, are the true descendants of paleolithic humans for whom physical activity was a must to survive in the harsh paleolithic era. What could be more beneficial to these descendants (athletes) than a diet that their ancestors ate for tens of thousands of years ?

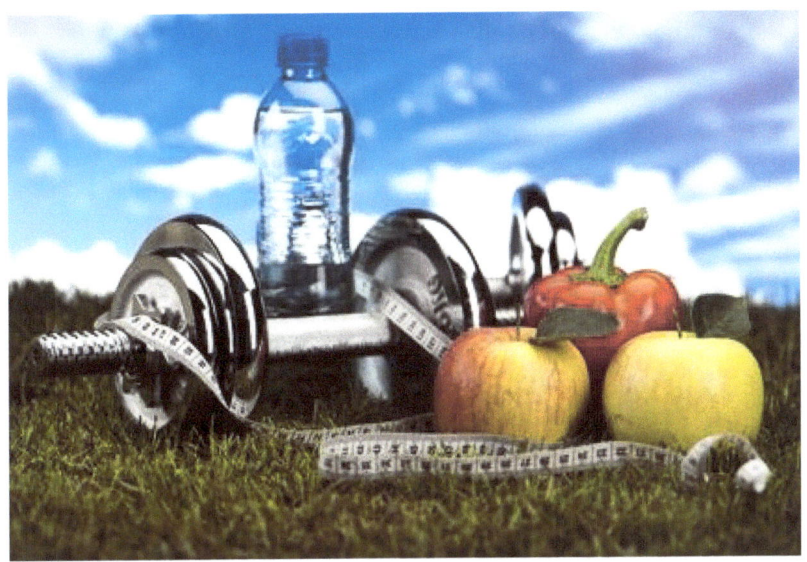

Dr. Loren Cordain and Joe Friel published a book titled **"The paleo diet for athletes"** in 2005 in which they attempted to prove that paleolithic diet is indeed the best diet for athletes. They highlighted the following benefits of paleo diet for athletes :

1. Paleo diet increases the intake of amino acids which have branched chains. This increases muscle development.
2. The stone age diet decreases the amount of omega-6 to omega-3 fatty acid ratio.
3. It lowers body acidity.
4. It is high in trace nutrients which facilitate in long term recovery from exercise.

In their own words :

"… the Paleo diet provides two benefits sought by all athletes : quick recovery for next workout, and superior health for the rest of your life."

Loren Cordain and Joe Friel: The paleo diet for athletes[8]

Hence, paleo diet is claimed to be the best dietary program for all people in general and for athletes in particular because it helps them achieve higher levels of health, fitness and strength. It has the ability to return humans to the same level of physical prowess, that their ancestors had while hunting stags and bisons, every other day.

Section II – Arguments against paleo diet

Despite all the research by paleo diet proponents to prove paleo diet to be the most effective diet, the question of paleo diet's efficacy is far from being answered. Several objections have been raised against paleo diet. Researchers have challenged the evolutionary logic behind paleo diet. Others have attempted to discredit the claim that paleo diet is the solution for modern diseases. It is said that the only reason that paleolithic ancestors didn't suffer from modern diseases was simply because their lives were too short and ended in youth, while these diseases mostly occur in adulthood. Several others have disputed the nature of the actual diet of human ancestors and concluded that our ancestors mostly ate plants instead of animals. All these arguments and some others are discussed in detail in this section.

Argument 1 : Did our ancestors really eat paleo ?

The first and most compelling argument that appears against paleo diet challenges its very foundations. The paleo diet proponents today advocate that humans of the stone age used to eat a high-protein, low-carbohydrate diet. But do we really know for sure what our ancestors ate ? No, not at all. The modern versions of the diet have been based on assumptions and some archeological evidence from Europe. Moreover, several researchers have suggested that a high-protein diet was not the actual diet of paleolithic humans. So, there are two important questions when the nature of the diet consumed by human ancestors is considered :

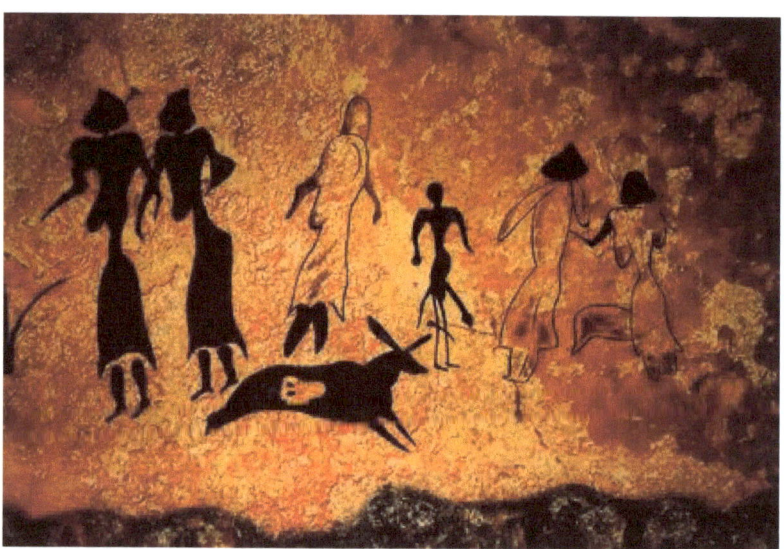

1. **What did our ancestors actually eat?** If we don't know exactly
    what our ancestors ate and in addition, if it is impossible to find out
    or prove what they ate, how can a specific diet plan be advocated to
    be paleolithic in the first place ? Whether the original evolutionary

hypothesis is right or wrong seems to be made irrelevant if we can't even determine what the diet of our ancestors actually was.

Starch Hypothesis: John McDougall has suggested in his book **"The Starch solution"** that humans of the paleolithic era didn't eat a high-protein diet ; rather they ate starch-based foods derived from the plants that were abundant in that era. [9]

Wheat may have been the staple food as early as 200,000 years ago: Another fact of great interest is that while all modern paleo diet programs strictly forbid the use of wheat and grains, Denis Murphy in his book **"People, plants and genes"** indicates that in some parts of the world, wheat was the staple food as early as 200,000 years ago ![10] This puts to test paleo diet proponents' assertion that agricultural foods such as wheat and grains appeared only 10,000 years ago.

Did our ancestors really eat the "paleo diet" which is so popular today? We may never know the answer.

2. **Did all humans of paleolithic era eat the same food?** Just as there is a wide cultural divergence today all over the world, is it not possible, rather likely that in the past there were all sorts of cultures in the world ? Could all of these people have similar diets ? The archeological evidence favoring high-protein diet is based in Europe. Even if we agree that a high-protein diet was eaten by Europeans, can we say with confidence that all over the world, humans ate the same diet ?

The Kung people: The wide cultural divergence among the primitive society is nowhere better demonstrated than in today's hunter-gatherer societies. Kung people of Africa today eat a diet that contains mostly plants (67 percent) while Canadian Eskimos eat a diet that is based solely on meat of wild animals.[11] It is likely that primitive hunter-gatherer societies showed the same divergence in their diets.

So, did our ancestors really eat the "paleo diet" which is so popular today? We may never know the exact answer.

Argument 2 : The evolutionary theory challenged.

The theory that human genome is adapted to the diet of the paleolithic era itself has been disputed. It is the fundamental concept in the paleo theory, that human genome continually adapted to stone age nutrition for around 2 million years and that humans have had insufficient time in the past 10,000 years to adapt to agricultural products. Two objections have been raised to this concept :

1. **Human genome isn't adapted to paleo diet:** Alexander Strohle and his colleagues at University of Hanover have disputed the adaptation of human genome to diet of stone age era. They state that the paleolithic theory considers genes to be the center of evolution i.e. it advocates the gene-centered evolutionary theory.

    According to Alexander Strohle, genes are independent of the diet humans take.

2. They believe that this theory is unproven. In their article **"Carbohydrates and the diet–atherosclerosis connection—More between earth and heaven"** they say that there is no one-to-one relation between genotype and phenotype.[12] Thus, the contention that human nutrition during that era left permanent effects on his genome is false. Rather, genes are independent of the diet humans take.

According to Katherine Milton, professor of physical anthropology at the University of California, human genome was formed, far before the hunter-gatherer era of history and whatever humans ate during paleolithic era had little, if any, effect on human genome.

".... (humans have) an evolutionary history as anthropoid primates stretching back more than 25 million years, a history that shaped their nutrient requirements and digestive physiology well before they were humans...." [11]

3. **10,000 years and still no adaptation?** The postulate that 10,000 years is too little time for adaptation is disputed by many scientists. Alexander Strohle et al argue that there have been more than 400-500 human generations since the advent of agriculture. If the diet of agriculturalists was in discordance with their genes and physiology, it would have created selection pressures, resulting in adequate adaptation to agriculture by now.

   Moreover, in recent history, there have been several examples of adaptations to diet such as development of lactose tolerance and increase in salivary amylase in humans. So, even if agricultural diet wasn't suited to human genome, by now, adaptations have made it quite suitable.

Argument 3 : The solution for all diseases ?

Several questions have been raised regarding the therapeutic value of paleo diet that is claimed by proponents of paleo diet. These arguments are discussed in the following text :

1. **Short brutal lives vs. long comfortable lives :** It is interesting to note that the average life span of our stone age ancestors, who are presented as models of health for us, was simply 20-24 years. Very few people got past that age. In comparison, humans today live 60 years on average. So, it is suggested that the reason chronic diseases didn't appear in stone age humans was simply because these are diseases of old age and humans in that era never reached this age.

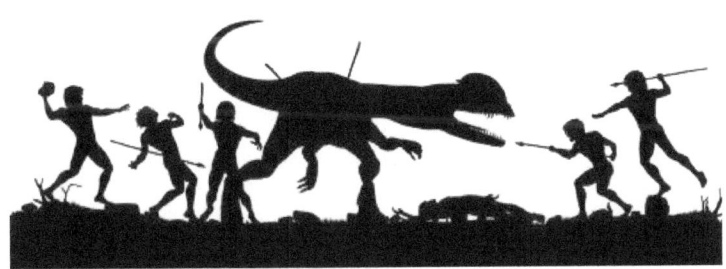

2. **Paleo diet or paleo physical activity?** Katherine Milton and several others have pointed out that the non-existence of diseases in hunter-gatherer societies doesn't have anything to do with their diets. She says that in the modern hunter-gatherer societies, there is wide disparity among the diets they consume.

Our stone age ancestors who are presented as models of health for us, lived on average for **20-24 years** !

3. On one hand, African Kung people consume a plant diet, while Canadian Eskimos consume solely meat. Yet, people of both these societies don't suffer from chronic diseases. The real reason for this is their activity level. Humans of modern societies lead sedentary lives, in which their diet easily exceeds their energy requirements, hunter-gatherers have have a high level of physical activity and consequently, a high energy requirement. Their diet never exceeds their energy requirement. She says :

   "In conclusion, it is likely that no hunter-gatherer society, regardless of the proportion of macronutrients consumed, suffered from diseases of civilization."[11]

4. **What about arthritis?** Despite the lack of many chronic diseases in hunter-gatherer societies, the one disease that is common in all these societies is arthritis, inflammation of joints. The reason is that the diet of these societies lacks calcium and essential vitamins as discussed in next section.

Argument 4 : The perfect diet or just another fad diet ?

While the paleo diet has been colored as a diet perfect for health promotion and disease prevention, it is far from perfect. Some have even gone so far to call paleo diet a "fad diet". Consuming paleo diet has several drawbacks which are not seen with eating modern diet. These drawbacks and shortcomings of paleo diet are detailed below :

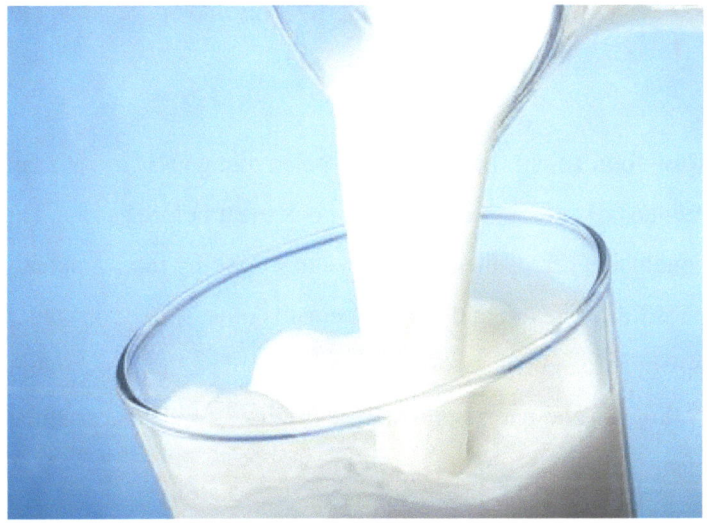

1. **Lack of essential nutrients :** The paleo diet suggested today consists almost totally of proteins and fats. It ignores many essential components of the diet such as vitamins and minerals. These ignored components include :
   - **Vitamin A**
   - **Vitamin C**
   - **Calcium**

- **Magnesium**
- **Iron**

Moreover, dairy products, which are essential source of calcium are restricted. This causes a deficiency of calcium which is responsible for several bone disorders such as arthritis (as mentioned in the previous argument).

2. **Saturated fat :** Beef and meat of other livestock animals, suggested in paleo diet programs, is often rich in saturated fat. This kind of fat has been proven to be harmful to humans and aggravates, rather than cures diseases such as atherosclerosis.

3. **Raw food :** Some proponents of paleo diet go so far as to say that humans of paleolithic era didn't cook meat before eating. This conclusion drives them to believe that cooking food is actually harmful for health and that raw meat is most suited for humans. This, however, can be hazardous as raw meat of cattle may contain several pathogens and parasites which cause diseases. These organisms are easily killed by simple cooking.

Thus, far from the perfect diets that they are painted to be, modern day paleo diets may actually be harmful in some ways.

Argument 5 : The 2011 study – The worst in 20 diets

In 2011, a team of US News and World Report evaluated different diets based on several factors including health, weight loss and ease of following. This team consisted of 22 experts. It is ironic that the rank of paleo diets among these 20 diets was 20th![13] The very last! It was ranked the least effective of all the diets for health promotion and weight loss.

In 2011, a report published by US News and World Report ranked paleo diet as the last in an analysis of 20 US diets!

In another 2012 survey, a diet based on Dukan diet was ranked lowest among 29 US diets. The survey concluded that :

"our experts took issue with the diet on every measure."

Dr. Loren Cordain responded by saying that as many as 5 studies have found paleo diet to be highly effective for weight loss and diabetes. The US News and World Report editors replied that they had reviewed those studies but had found them to be too short to draw any strong conclusions.

Conclusion : A 10,000 year old dispute – The tribe leader and the old man

In conclusion, it seems that researchers today are in disagreement regarding the effectiveness of paleo diet. In your imagination (see Introduction), the tribe leader and the old man had different views regarding agriculture; the tribe leader sought something new and the old man wanted to uphold the traditions of old. This dispute seems to be unresolved even today, 10,000 years later.

What was the diet of our ancestors? Is it really better than modern diet ? Although the answer to these questions isn't clear, this much is clear : The modern diet and life style have created many problems for humans. Sedentary lifestyle and overeating seem to be the culprits behind today's diseases.   Going back to the same level of physical activity as our ancestors and eating paleo diet sensibly and adding certain foods such as dairy products which are deficient in paleo diet may be the best method to avoid modern diseases.

Paleo diet has its positives and negatives. However, more research is needed before a solid verdict can be given in favor or against paleo diet. But as you open your eyes in this modern era, what do you think ? After taking this scientific trip through the stone age, will you continue to eat as you always have or will you make sure that all the unhealthy foods keep out of your diet so that you achieve the maximum fitness that you are capable of ? Your health, your fitness and your diet ; all these things are in your hand.

References

1. Walter Voegtlin: The Stone age diet based on in-depth study of Human ecology and diet of man (1975) – CHAPTER 15: A 20th Century Stone age diet (http://www.mitodascalorias.com/wp-content/uploads/2013/06/Voegtlin_1975_The_Stone_Age_Diet.pdf)

2. Wikipedia's definition of Paleolithic diet (http://en.wikipedia.org/wiki/Paleolithic_diet)

3. Walter Voegtlin: The Stone age diet based on in-depth study of Human ecology and diet of man (1975) (http://www.mitodascalorias.com/wp-content/uploads/2013/06/Voegtlin_1975_The_Stone_Age_Diet.pdf)

4. Boyd Eaton, Loren Cordain, Staffan Lindeberg: Evolutionary Health Promotions: A consideration of common counterarguments. December, 2001. (http://thepaleodiet.com/wp-content/uploads/2012/04/Counter-Arguments-Paper.pdf)

5. Boyd Eaton: Paleolithic nutrition – A consideration of its nature and current implications 1985 (http://www.ncbi.nlm.nih.gov/pubmed/2981409?dopt=Abstract)

6. Gary Foster et al. A randomized trial of a Low Carbohydrate diet for Obesity. (http://inspire.stat.ucla.edu/unit_15/NEJM2082.pdf)

7. Staffan Lindeberg et al. Apparent absence of stroke and ischaemic heart disease in a traditional Melanesian island: a clinical study in Kitava.
(http://onlinelibrary.wiley.com/doi/10.1111/j.1365-2796.1993.tb00986.x/abstract;jsessionid=7F1EEC9B23FCAD9333A2D12078313A4C.d02t01)

8. Loren Cordain and John Friel: The Paleo diet for athletes.
(http://www.trainingbible.com/pdf/Paleo_for_Athletes_Cliff_Notes.pdf)

9. Dr. John McDougall: The Starch Solution
(http://www.drmcdougall.com/store_starch_solution.html)

10. Dr. Denis Murphy: People, plants and genes – The Story of Crops and Humanity.
(http://www.oxfordscholarship.com/view/10.1093/acprof:oso/9780199207145.001.0001/acprof-9780199207145)

11. Katherine Milton: Hunter-gatherer diets – a different perspective
(http://ajcn.nutrition.org/content/71/3/665.long)

12. Alexander Strohle et al.: Carbohydrates and the diet-atherosclerosis connection--more between earth and heaven. Comment on the article "The atherogenic potential of dietary carbohydrate".
(http://scholar.qsensei.com/content/1321gb
http://www.ncbi.nlm.nih.gov/pubmed/16997359)

13. US. News and World Reports 2012 – Best overall diets
    (http://health.usnews.com/best-diet/best-overall-diets)

Photo credits
All images licensed by fotolia.com

Human evolution vector

© *laci619 - Fotolia.com*

milk pouring into glass

© *Nitr - Fotolia.com*

Weight Loss Success

© *Mark Hayes - Fotolia.com*

Charles Darwin

© *nickolae - Fotolia.com*

Cave painting of primitive commune

© *Nomad_Soul - Fotolia.com*

Dna double helix molecules and chromosomes

© *nobeastsofierce - Fotolia.com*

Positives and Negatives

© *mwellis - Fotolia.com*

Prehistoric hunt

© *Adrian Hillman - Fotolia.com*

Vitamin and Fitness diet, green grass

© *Sebastian Duda - Fotolia.com*

Cooked Beef Roast

© *portokalis - Fotolia.com*

Cave painting of primitive hunt

© *Nomad_Soul - Fotolia.com*

Author Bio

Muhammad Usman is a distinguished medical graduate of Allama iqbal medical college (AIMC). He is a professional writer who has been in the field for more than 4 years. During this time he has produced 10,000+ articles, blogs and eBooks on various niches related to diseases, health, fitness, nutrition and well-being. He is a regular contributor to several journals related to medicine and surgery. He is the editor of several journals and newspapers.

Check out some of the other JD-Biz Publishing books

Gardening Series on Amazon

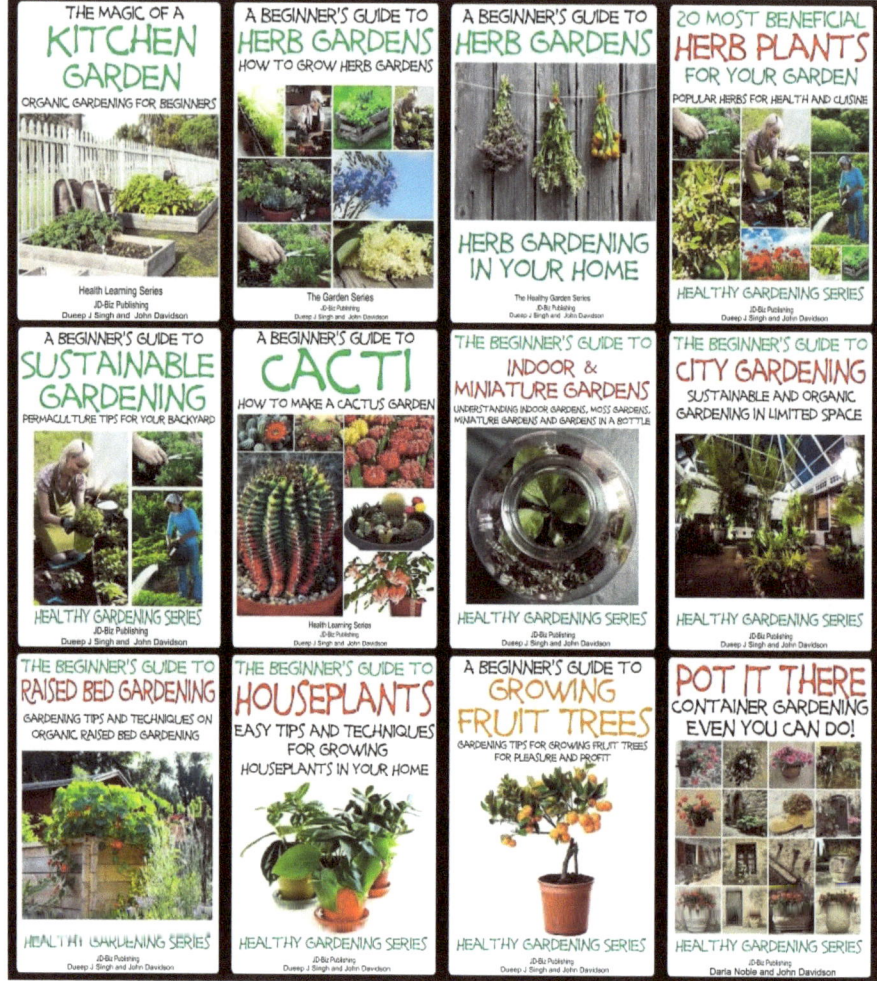

Download Free Books!
http://MendonCottageBooks.com

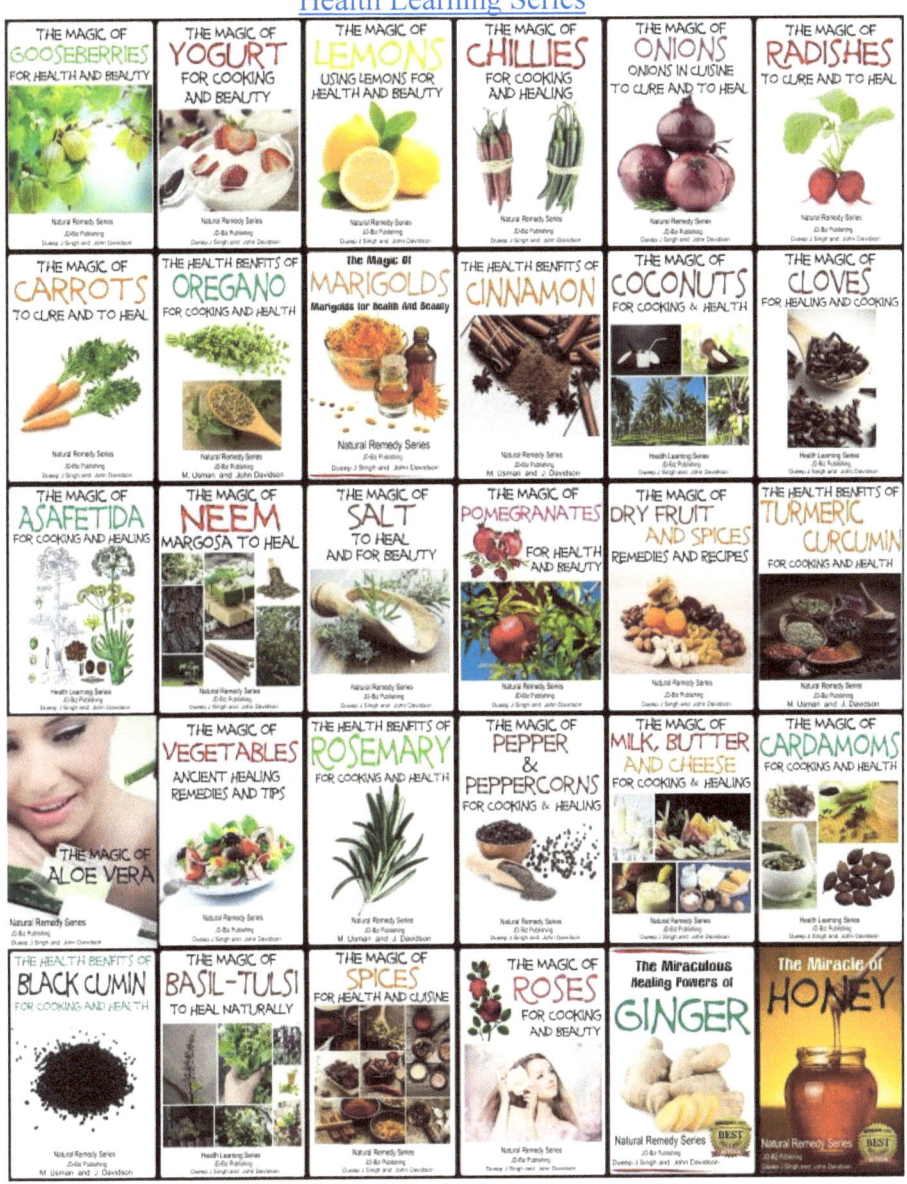

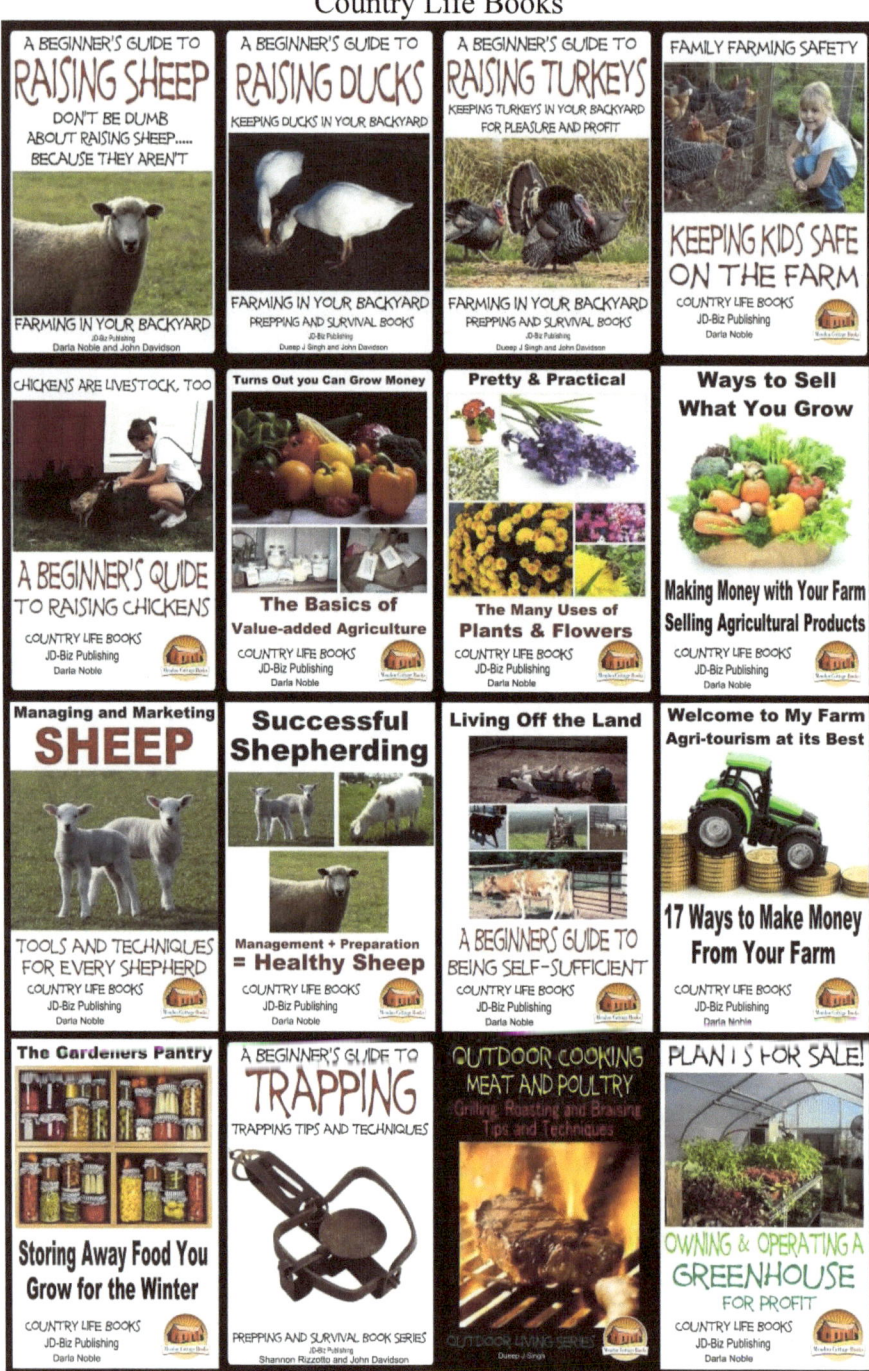

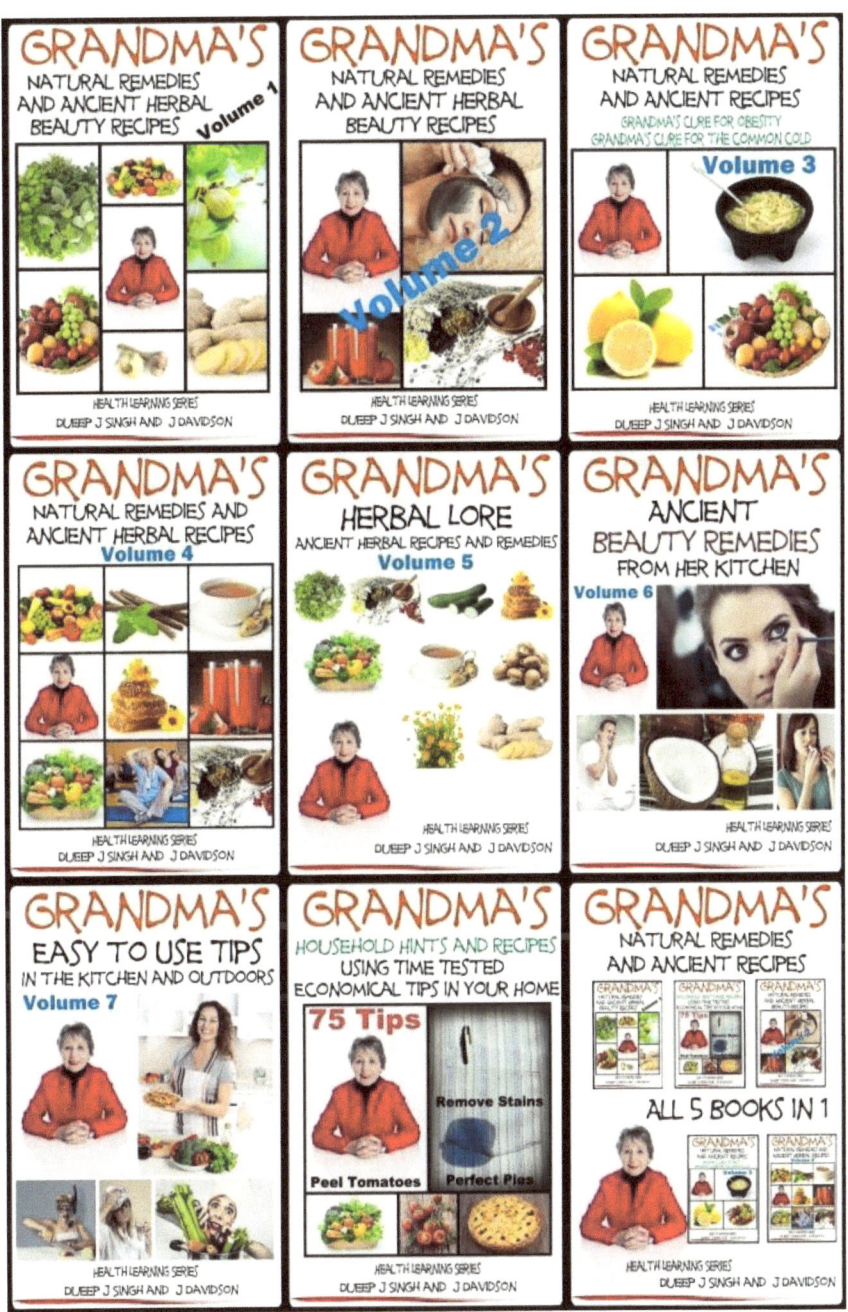

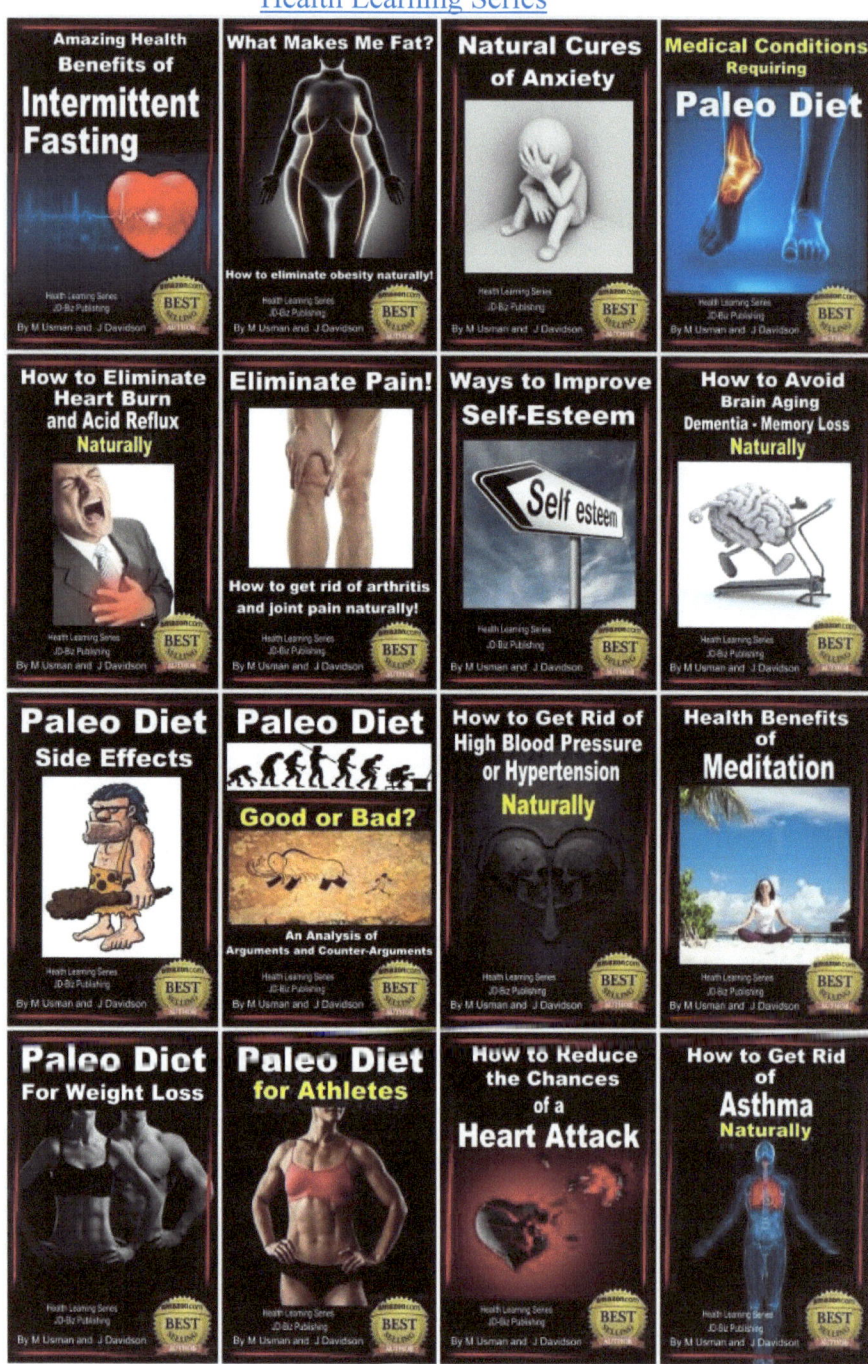

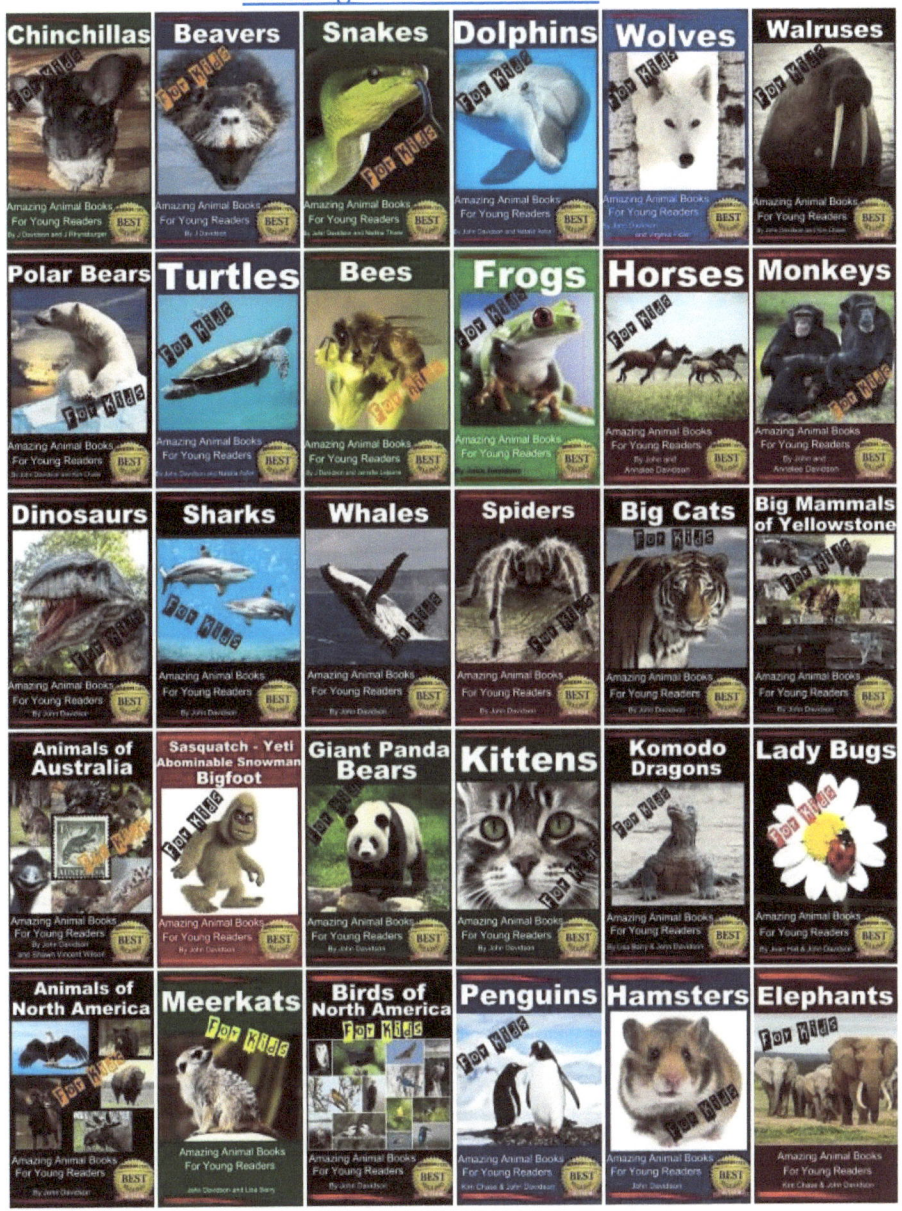

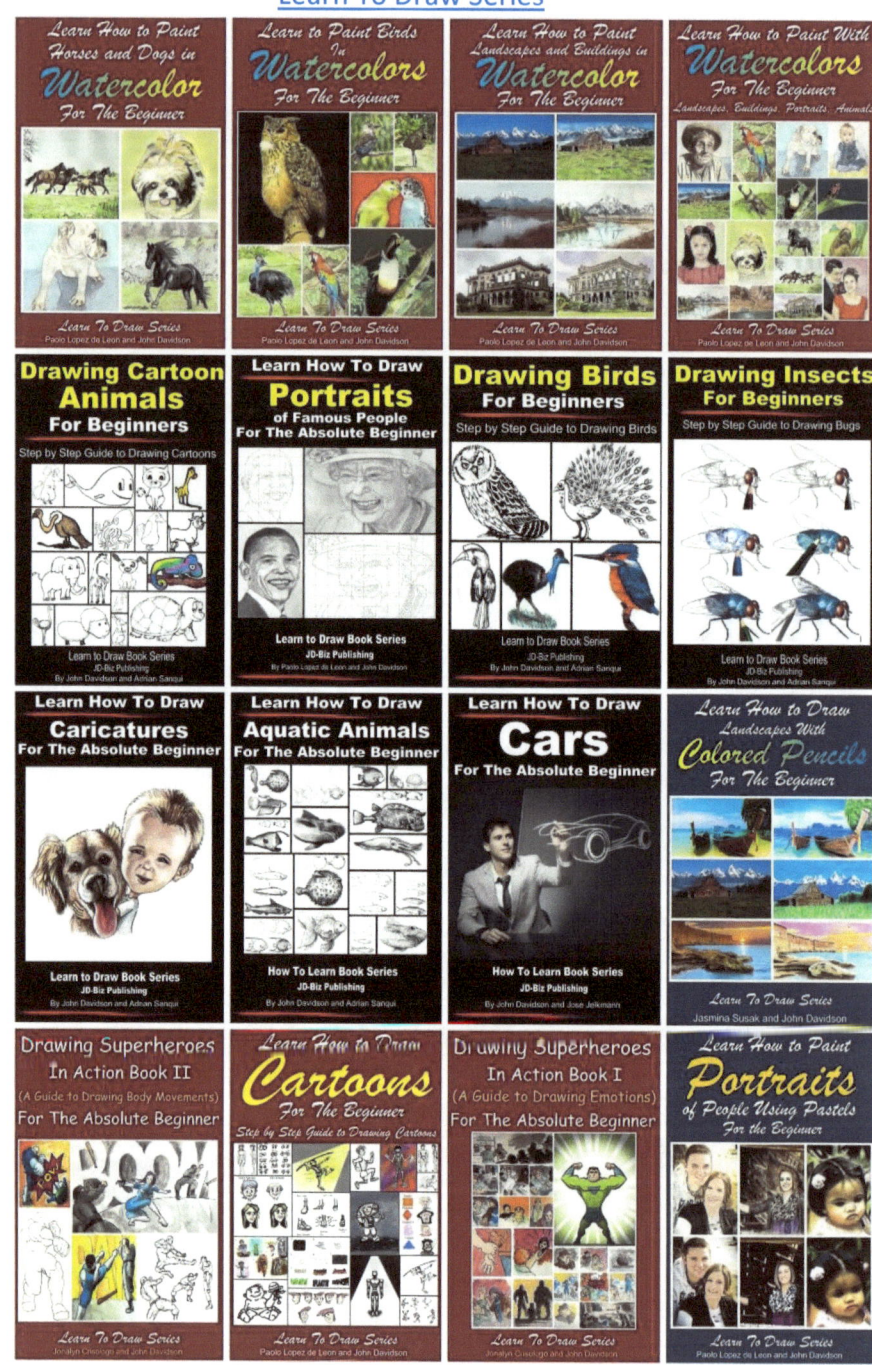

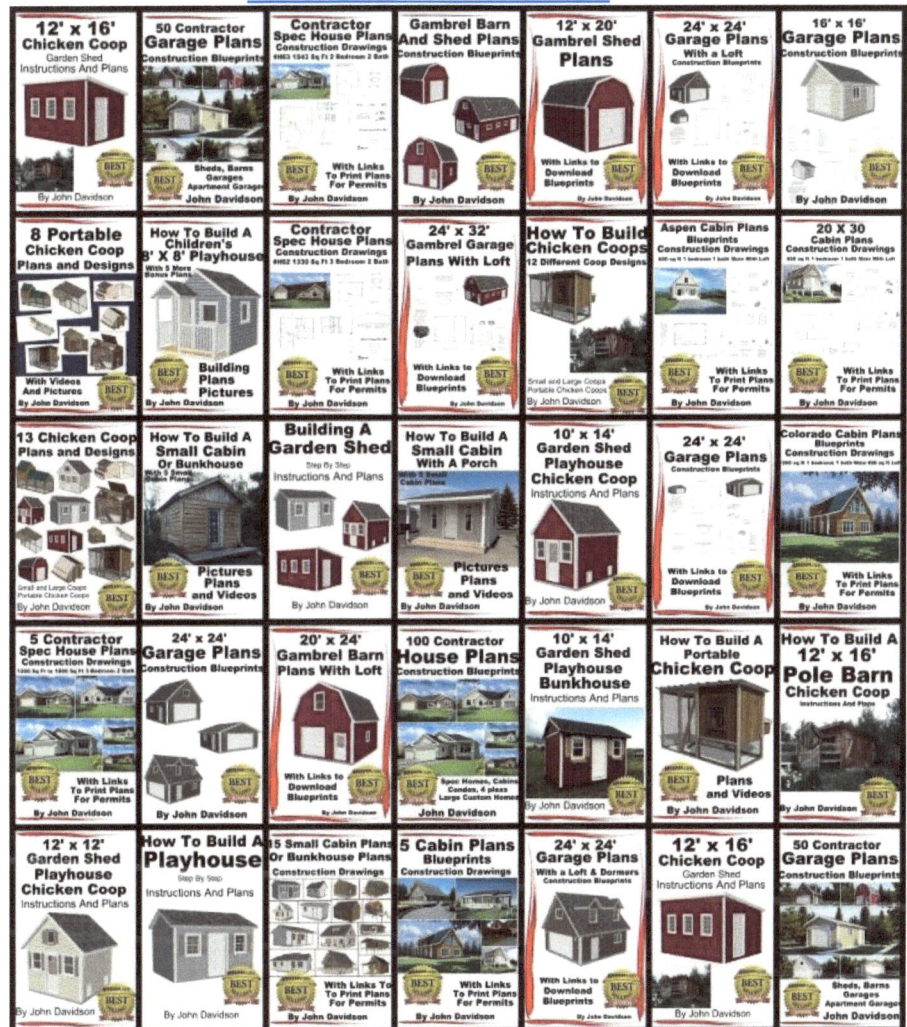

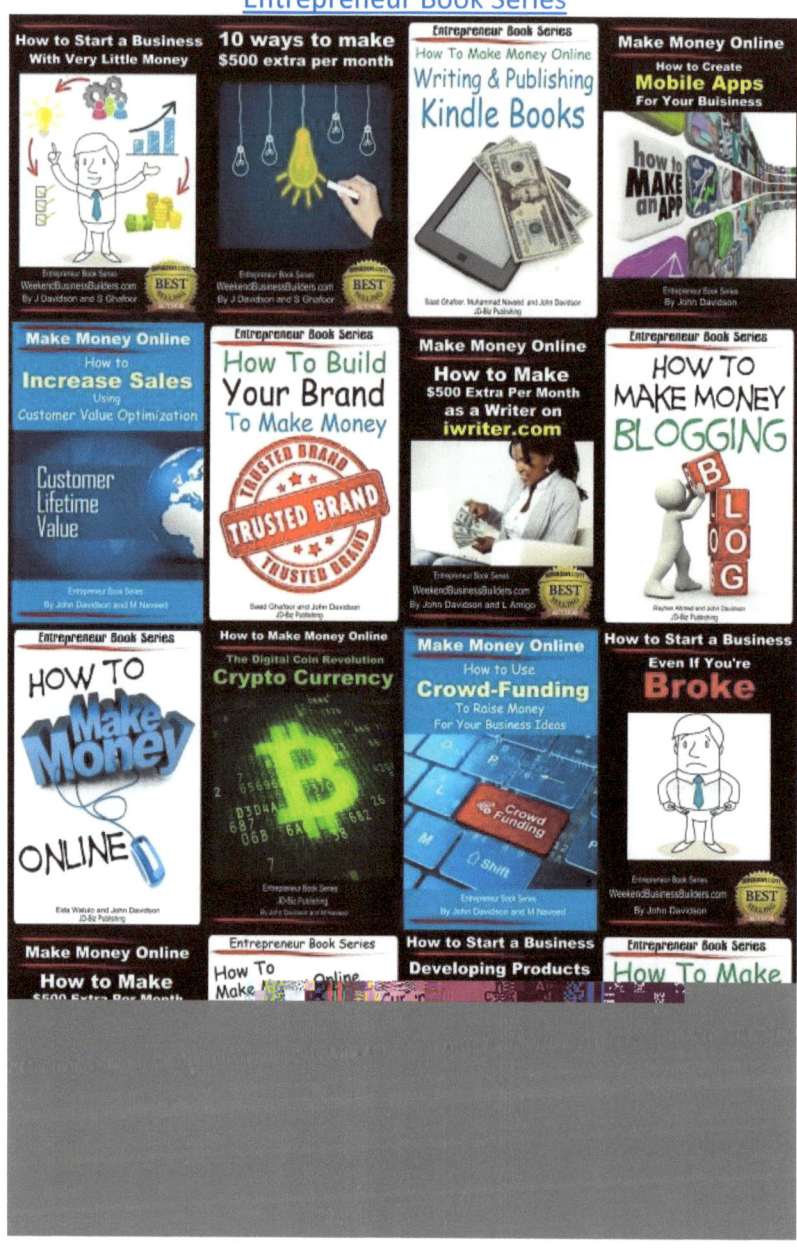

Our books are available at

1. Amazon.com
2. Barnes and Noble
3. Itunes
4. Kobo
5. Smashwords
6. Google Play Books

Download Free Books!
http://MendonCottageBooks.com

Publisher

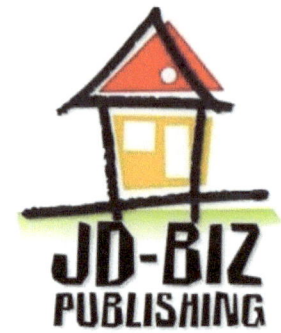

JD-Biz Corp

P O Box 374

Mendon, Utah 84325

http://www.jd-biz.com/

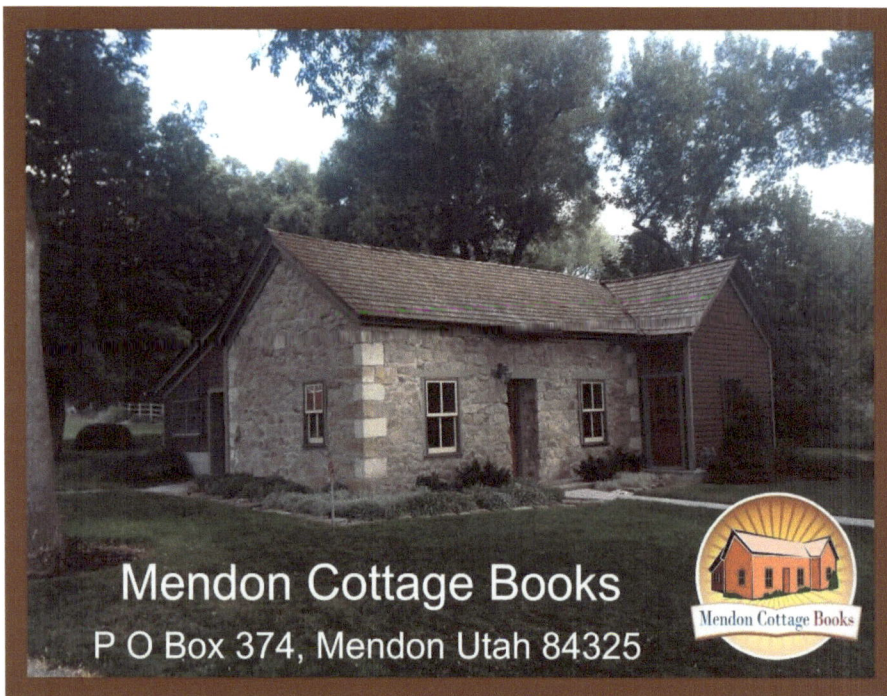

Mendon Cottage Books

P O Box 374, Mendon Utah 84325

www.ingramcontent.com/pod-product-compliance
Lightning Source LLC
Chambersburg PA
CBHW050833290526
45792CB00001B/375